THE EARLY SIGNS OF PREGNANCY YOU MIGHT NOT KNOW ABOUT

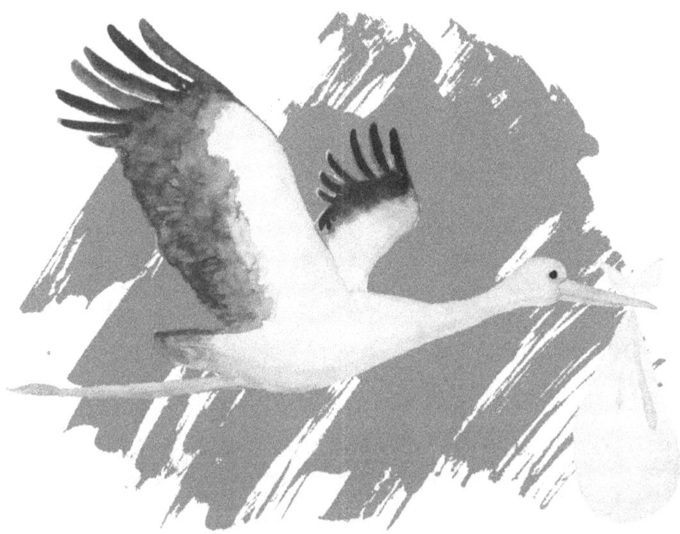

Aurora Brooks

xspurts.com

Created by <u>BabyDreamers.net</u>

Free Book Offer:
<u>Get How to be a Super Mom For Free</u>

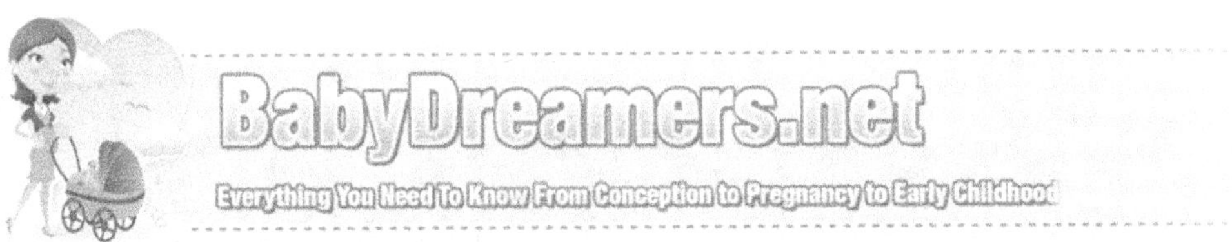

A Short Read is a type of book that is designed to be read in one quick sitting.

These no fluff books are perfect for people who want an overview about a subject in a short period of time.

Table of Contents

CHANGES IN SALIVA

INCREASED THIRST

SKIN DARKENING

FREQUENTLY ASKED QUESTIONS

Have Questions / Comments?

Get How To Be A Super Mom 100% FREE

The Early Signs of Pregnancy You Might Not Know About

The early signs of pregnancy can vary from woman to woman and may not always be the most obvious indicators. While a missed period or positive pregnancy test are commonly known signs, there are several lesser-known symptoms that women may experience before these milestones. These early signs can provide valuable insights into the possibility of pregnancy and help women recognize the changes happening in their bodies.

One of the early signs of pregnancy is breast changes. Many women experience tenderness, swelling, and darkening of the nipples during the early stages of pregnancy. These changes occur due to hormonal fluctuations and increased blood flow to the breasts. Paying attention to these subtle changes can provide a clue that pregnancy may be underway.

Another early sign to watch out for is increased urination. Hormonal changes during pregnancy can affect the bladder, leading to more frequent trips to the bathroom. If you find yourself needing to urinate more often than usual, it could be an indication that you are pregnant.

Changes in vaginal discharge can also be an early sign of pregnancy. Some women may notice an increase in the amount of discharge or a change in consistency. These changes occur as a result of increased blood flow to the vaginal area and the body's preparation for pregnancy.

Spotting or light bleeding, known as implantation bleeding, can occur when the fertilized egg attaches to the uterine lining. This can be mistaken for a light period, but it is actually an early pregnancy symptom. If you experience light bleeding around the time your period is due, it may be worth considering the possibility of pregnancy.

Heightened sense of smell or aversion to certain odors can also be an early sign of pregnancy. Many pregnant women find that they become more sensitive to smells during the early stages. Certain odors that were once tolerable may suddenly become overwhelming or even nauseating.

Fatigue is a common symptom experienced by many women in the early stages of pregnancy. Hormonal changes and increased energy demands can leave you feeling extremely tired. If you find yourself needing more rest than usual or feeling exhausted even after a good night's sleep, it could be a sign that you are pregnant.

Morning sickness, although widely known, is still an important early sign of pregnancy. It refers to the nausea and vomiting that many pregnant women experience, particularly in the first trimester. While it is called "morning" sickness, it can actually occur at any time of the day.

Food cravings and aversions are also common in early pregnancy. Many women develop strong desires for specific foods or may suddenly find themselves repulsed by foods they once enjoyed. These cravings and aversions are thought to be influenced by hormonal changes.

Mood swings and emotional changes are another early sign of pregnancy. Hormonal fluctuations can affect neurotransmitters in the brain, leading to changes in mood and emotional sensitivity. It's not uncommon for pregnant women to experience a rollercoaster of emotions during the early stages.

Constipation is a common symptom due to hormonal changes affecting the digestive system. The slowing down of the digestive process can result in difficulty passing stools. Staying hydrated, eating fiber-rich foods, and engaging in regular physical activity can help alleviate this symptom.

Headaches can also be a symptom of early pregnancy. Hormonal changes and increased blood volume can lead to headaches. If you experience frequent headaches, it may be worth considering the possibility of pregnancy.

Feelings of dizziness and lightheadedness can occur in early pregnancy. These symptoms can be attributed to hormonal changes and increased blood flow. Taking frequent breaks, staying hydrated, and avoiding sudden movements can help manage these symptoms.

A heightened sense of smell is another early sign of pregnancy. Certain smells may become more intense and may even trigger nausea. This sensitivity to smells can be quite strong during the early stages of pregnancy.

Acne breakouts and skin changes can also occur in early pregnancy. Hormonal changes can lead to an increase in oil production, resulting in acne breakouts. Some women may also notice changes in their skin, such as darkening of the linea nigra (a line that forms on the abdomen) or darkened underarms.

Changes in libido can vary from woman to woman during early pregnancy. Some women may experience an increase in sexual desire, while others may experience a decrease. These changes are influenced by hormonal fluctuations and can be temporary.

Abdominal bloating and gas are common early pregnancy symptoms. Hormonal changes can slow down digestion, leading to bloating and discomfort. Eating smaller, more frequent meals and avoiding gas-producing foods can help alleviate these symptoms.

Tracking your basal body temperature can help detect early pregnancy. A slight increase in basal body temperature can indicate that ovulation has occurred and fertilization may have taken place.

Some women may experience nasal congestion and stuffiness in early pregnancy. Hormonal changes can cause the blood vessels in the nasal passages to swell, leading to congestion. Using saline nasal sprays and staying hydrated can help alleviate these symptoms.

Changes in saliva consistency and taste can also be an early sign of pregnancy. Some women may notice an increase in saliva production or a change in taste. These changes are thought to be influenced by hormonal fluctuations.

Increased thirst can be an early sign of pregnancy. Hormonal changes can affect fluid balance in the body, leading to increased thirst. Staying hydrated is important during pregnancy, so be sure to drink plenty of water.

Hormonal changes can cause skin darkening in early pregnancy. The linea nigra, a dark line that forms on the abdomen, is a common example of this. Some women may also notice darkening of the underarms or other areas of the body.

These are just a few of the early signs of pregnancy that women may experience before a missed period or positive pregnancy test. It's important to remember that every woman is different, and not all women will experience the same symptoms. If you suspect you may be pregnant, it's always best to consult with a healthcare professional for confirmation.

Breast Changes

During early pregnancy, many women experience noticeable changes in their breasts. These changes can occur even before a missed period or positive pregnancy test.

Understanding these common breast changes can help you recognize the early signs of pregnancy.

One of the most common breast changes in early pregnancy is breast tenderness. Your breasts may feel more sensitive or sore to the touch. This tenderness is caused by hormonal changes in your body as it prepares for pregnancy. It is important to note that breast tenderness can also be a symptom of premenstrual syndrome (PMS), so it is essential to consider other early pregnancy signs as well.

In addition to tenderness, you may also notice swelling in your breasts. This swelling is caused by increased blood flow and hormonal changes. Your breasts may feel fuller and heavier than usual. The increase in size and weight can be uncomfortable, but it is a normal part of early pregnancy.

Another breast change that can occur in early pregnancy is darkening of the nipples. Your nipples may become darker and more prominent due to hormonal fluctuations. This is known as the areolas darkening. It is a natural process that prepares your breasts for breastfeeding. Some women may also notice small bumps on the areolas, known as Montgomery's tubercles.

It is important to remember that every woman's experience with breast changes in early pregnancy can vary. Some women may experience all of these changes, while others may only notice one or two. If you suspect you may be pregnant and are experiencing breast changes, it is recommended to take a pregnancy test and consult with your healthcare provider for confirmation.

Increased Urination

One of the lesser-known early signs of pregnancy is increased urination. Many women may notice that they need to urinate more frequently than usual, even before they miss a period or take a pregnancy test. This symptom can be attributed to hormonal changes that occur during pregnancy.

During pregnancy, the body produces more human chorionic gonadotropin (hCG) hormone, which can affect the bladder. The increased levels of hCG can result in increased blood flow to the pelvic area and kidneys, leading to increased urine production. Additionally, as the uterus expands, it can put pressure on the bladder, causing the need to urinate more frequently.

It is important to stay hydrated during pregnancy, so drinking plenty of water is essential. However, it may be helpful to avoid excessive fluid intake close to bedtime to minimize nighttime bathroom trips. It is also recommended to empty the bladder completely each time to reduce the risk of urinary tract infections.

Changes in Vaginal Discharge

Changes in vaginal discharge can be one of the early signs of pregnancy that many women may experience. It is important to understand how these changes can indicate early pregnancy. During pregnancy, hormonal fluctuations can affect the vaginal discharge, leading to an increased amount and different consistency.

One of the changes that women may notice is an increase in the amount of vaginal discharge. This is due to an increase in blood flow to the vaginal area, which stimulates the glands to produce more discharge. The discharge may also become thicker and stickier than usual.

In addition to the increase in amount, the consistency of the vaginal discharge may also change. It may become milky or creamy in texture. Some women may also notice a slight yellow or white color to the discharge.

These changes in vaginal discharge are a result of the hormonal changes that occur during early pregnancy. The increased amount and different consistency of the discharge can be a sign that the body is preparing for pregnancy and the changes that will occur in the reproductive system.

It is important to note that changes in vaginal discharge can also be caused by other factors, such as infections or hormonal imbalances. If you are experiencing any unusual or concerning symptoms, it is always best to consult with a healthcare professional for a proper diagnosis.

Spotting or Light Bleeding

Implantation bleeding is a common early pregnancy symptom that can often be mistaken for a light period. It occurs when the fertilized egg implants itself into the uterine lining, causing some minor bleeding. This usually happens around 6-12 days after conception, which is around the time when a woman would expect her period. However, implantation bleeding is usually much lighter and shorter in duration than a regular period.

Spotting or light bleeding during early pregnancy can be a sign that the fertilized egg has successfully implanted in the uterus. The bleeding is usually light pink or brown in color and may only last for a day or two. Some women may mistake this bleeding for their period and not realize that they are actually pregnant.

It's important to note that not all women will experience implantation bleeding, and its presence or absence does not necessarily indicate a problem with the pregnancy. However, if you do experience any bleeding during early pregnancy, it's always a good idea to consult with your healthcare provider to rule out any potential complications.

Changes in Sense of Smell

Discover how heightened sense of smell or aversion to certain odors can be an early sign of pregnancy.

One of the lesser-known early signs of pregnancy is a change in sense of smell. Many women experience a heightened sense of smell during the early stages of pregnancy. Suddenly, everyday smells that were once pleasant or neutral may become overpowering and even nauseating. This change in olfactory perception can be attributed to the hormonal changes that occur in the body.

Some women may also develop aversions to certain odors that they previously enjoyed. For example, the smell of coffee or cooking meat may suddenly become unbearable. This aversion to certain smells can be a strong indicator that a woman is pregnant.

It is believed that this heightened sense of smell and aversion to certain odors serves as a protective mechanism for the developing fetus. Certain odors, such as those associated with spoiled or harmful substances, may trigger a negative response in order to prevent the pregnant woman from consuming anything potentially harmful.

If you find yourself suddenly repulsed by certain smells or noticing scents that others don't seem to detect, it may be worth considering the possibility of pregnancy. Of course, changes in sense of smell can vary from woman to woman, so it's important to remember that not everyone will experience this particular symptom.

It's also worth noting that changes in sense of smell can occur for reasons other than pregnancy, such as hormonal fluctuations or certain medical conditions. Therefore, it's always a good idea to consult with a healthcare professional if you suspect you may be pregnant or if you have any concerns about changes in your sense of smell.

Fatigue

Fatigue is a common symptom experienced by many women in the early stages of pregnancy. It is a feeling of extreme tiredness and lack of energy that can make even the simplest tasks feel exhausting. This fatigue is often attributed to the hormonal changes that occur in the body during pregnancy.

During early pregnancy, the body undergoes significant hormonal fluctuations as it prepares for the growth and development of the baby. These hormonal changes can have a profound impact on a woman's energy levels. The increased production of progesterone, for example, can cause feelings of drowsiness and lethargy.

In addition to hormonal changes, the body also experiences increased energy demands during early pregnancy. The growing fetus requires a significant amount of energy for its development, and this can leave the mother feeling depleted. The body redirects energy resources to support the baby's growth, which can leave the mother feeling fatigued.

To manage fatigue during early pregnancy, it is important to prioritize rest and self-care. Getting enough sleep and taking regular breaks throughout the day can help combat feelings of exhaustion. It is also important to eat a balanced diet and stay hydrated to support the body's energy needs. Gentle exercise, such as walking or prenatal yoga, can also help boost energy levels.

It is important to remember that fatigue is a normal part of early pregnancy and is usually temporary. However, if fatigue becomes overwhelming or is accompanied by other concerning symptoms, it is important to consult a healthcare provider for further evaluation.

Morning Sickness

Morning sickness is a classic symptom of pregnancy that many women experience in the early stages. Despite its name, morning sickness can occur at any time of the day or night. It is characterized by feelings of nausea and vomiting, which can range from mild to severe. While the exact cause of morning sickness is unknown, hormonal changes during pregnancy are believed to play a significant role.

One theory suggests that the rise in pregnancy hormones, such as human chorionic gonadotropin (hCG) and estrogen, may irritate the stomach lining, leading to feelings of nausea. Additionally, the sense of smell becomes heightened during pregnancy, and certain smells can trigger nausea and vomiting. The good news is that morning sickness usually subsides by the end of the first trimester.

If you're experiencing morning sickness, there are several tips that may help alleviate the symptoms:

- Eat small, frequent meals throughout the day to avoid an empty stomach.
- Avoid spicy, greasy, or strong-smelling foods that may trigger nausea.
- Stay hydrated by sipping on water, ginger ale, or herbal teas.
- Try eating bland, easily digestible foods like crackers, toast, or rice.
- Get plenty of rest and take breaks when needed.
- Consider trying natural remedies like ginger or acupressure wristbands.

It's important to remember that every pregnancy is different, and what works for one woman may not work for another. If your morning sickness is severe and interfering with your daily life, it's best to consult with your healthcare provider for further guidance and potential treatment options.

Food Cravings and Aversions

One of the most well-known and talked-about early signs of pregnancy is food cravings. Many pregnant women experience strong desires for specific foods, often ones they wouldn't normally eat. These cravings can range from the common, like pickles and ice cream, to the more unusual, like craving non-food items such as dirt or chalk. While the exact cause of food cravings during pregnancy is not fully understood, hormonal changes are believed to play a role.

On the flip side, some pregnant women may also experience food aversions, where they have a strong dislike or repulsion towards certain foods. This can be frustrating for expectant mothers who suddenly find themselves unable to stomach foods they once enjoyed. Again, hormonal changes are thought to be the culprit behind these aversions.

The reasons behind specific food cravings and aversions during pregnancy are still a mystery, but it's believed that they may be the body's way of ensuring the mother and baby receive the necessary nutrients. For example, cravings for salty foods may indicate a need for increased sodium intake, while aversions to certain strong-smelling foods may help protect the mother and baby from potential toxins.

It's important to note that while food cravings and aversions are common in pregnancy, they can vary greatly from woman to woman. Some may experience intense cravings and aversions, while others may not have any at all. It's also worth mentioning that cravings and aversions can change throughout the pregnancy, so what a woman craves or dislikes in the early stages may be different later on.

If you're experiencing food cravings or aversions during pregnancy, it's generally safe to indulge in your cravings as long as they are not harmful to you or your baby. However, it's important to maintain a balanced diet and make healthy choices whenever possible. If you have concerns about your cravings or aversions, it's always best to consult with your healthcare provider for guidance.

Mood Swings

Mood Swings

During early pregnancy, hormonal fluctuations can have a significant impact on a woman's mood and emotions. These hormonal changes, particularly the rise in estrogen and progesterone levels, can cause mood swings and emotional changes that may vary from woman to woman.

One moment, a pregnant woman may feel elated and excited about the upcoming journey of motherhood, and the next moment, she may find herself bursting into tears for no apparent reason. These rapid shifts in mood can be attributed to the hormonal roller coaster happening within her body.

It's important to remember that mood swings during early pregnancy are completely normal and a common experience for many women. The surge in hormones can affect neurotransmitters in the brain, leading to emotional ups and downs.

Dealing with mood swings during this time can be challenging, but there are strategies to help manage them. It's crucial for women to prioritize self-care and engage in activities that promote relaxation and stress reduction. This may include practicing mindfulness, engaging in gentle exercise, getting enough rest, and seeking support from loved ones.

Additionally, open communication with a healthcare provider can provide reassurance and guidance on managing mood swings during pregnancy. They may be able to offer coping strategies or recommend support groups or counseling services.

Remember, every woman's experience with mood swings during early pregnancy is unique, and it's essential to be patient and kind to oneself during this time of emotional adjustment.

Constipation

Constipation is a common early pregnancy symptom that many women experience. It occurs when the digestive system slows down due to hormonal changes in the body. During pregnancy, the hormone progesterone increases, which can relax the muscles in the intestines and cause them to move more slowly. This can lead to a buildup of waste material in the colon, resulting in difficulty passing stools.

There are several reasons why hormonal changes affect the digestive system and contribute to constipation. Firstly, progesterone can cause the muscles in the intestines to become less efficient at pushing waste through the digestive tract. Additionally, the growing uterus can put pressure on the intestines, further slowing down the movement of stool. Lastly, prenatal vitamins and iron supplements, which are commonly recommended during pregnancy, can also contribute to constipation.

To alleviate constipation during early pregnancy, there are several strategies you can try. Increasing your fiber intake by consuming fruits, vegetables, and whole grains can help soften the stool and promote regular bowel movements. Staying hydrated is also important, as drinking plenty of water can help prevent dehydration and keep the digestive system functioning properly. Regular exercise, such as walking or gentle yoga, can stimulate the muscles in the intestines and help relieve constipation.

In addition to these lifestyle changes, some women may find relief from over-the-counter stool softeners or laxatives. However, it is important to consult with a healthcare professional before taking any medication during pregnancy to ensure it is safe for both you and your baby.

Headaches

Headaches are a common symptom experienced by many women in early pregnancy. These headaches can range from mild to severe and can be quite bothersome. But what causes these headaches?

One possible cause of headaches in early pregnancy is hormonal changes. During pregnancy, there is a surge in hormones such as estrogen and progesterone, which can affect blood vessels and lead to headaches. Additionally, the increased blood volume in the body can also contribute to headaches.

Managing headaches during early pregnancy can be challenging, but there are some strategies that may help. It's important to stay hydrated and drink plenty of water throughout the day. Getting enough rest and practicing relaxation techniques, such as deep breathing or gentle stretching, can also provide relief. If the headaches persist or become severe, it's always best to consult with a healthcare provider for further evaluation and guidance.

Dizziness

Feeling dizzy or lightheaded can be a common symptom of early pregnancy. Hormonal changes, particularly a rise in progesterone levels, can affect blood circulation and lead to feelings of dizziness. Additionally, the expanding uterus can put pressure on blood vessels, further contributing to this symptom.

If you experience dizziness during early pregnancy, there are a few things you can do to manage it:

- Stay hydrated: Dehydration can worsen dizziness, so make sure to drink plenty of fluids throughout the day.
- Rise slowly: When getting up from a lying or sitting position, do so slowly to give your body time to adjust to changes in blood pressure.
- Eat regular meals: Low blood sugar levels can also contribute to dizziness, so try to eat small, frequent meals to keep your blood sugar stable.
- Avoid standing for long periods: Prolonged standing can exacerbate dizziness, so try to take breaks and sit down when possible.
- Wear loose, comfortable clothing: Tight clothing can restrict blood flow and contribute to dizziness, so opt for loose-fitting garments.

If your dizziness is severe or accompanied by other concerning symptoms, it's important to consult with your healthcare provider to rule out any underlying conditions.

Heightened Sense of Smell

During early pregnancy, many women experience a heightened sense of smell, which can be an early sign of pregnancy. This means that their sense of smell becomes more sensitive than usual, and they may notice smells more intensely than before. It's like having a superpower, but instead of being able to fly or lift heavy objects, you can detect even the faintest scent from miles away.

This heightened sense of smell can be both a blessing and a curse. On one hand, it can be enjoyable to appreciate the delightful aroma of freshly baked bread or the sweet scent of flowers. On the other hand, it can also be overwhelming and even nauseating when certain smells trigger a wave of morning sickness.

Speaking of morning sickness, the connection between a heightened sense of smell and nausea is quite strong. Many pregnant women find that certain smells, such as the aroma of cooking meat or the scent of strong perfumes, can make them feel queasy or even lead to vomiting. It's like their nose becomes a detective, sniffing out any potential threats to their sensitive stomach.

So why does this happen? Well, it's believed that hormonal changes during pregnancy play a significant role. The surge in hormones can affect the olfactory system, which is responsible for our sense of smell. This can lead to an increased sensitivity to odors, making certain smells more noticeable and potent.

It's important to note that the heightened sense of smell is not the same for every pregnant woman. Some may experience it more intensely than others, while some may not experience it at all. Every pregnancy is unique, and the symptoms can vary from woman to woman.

If you find that certain smells are triggering your morning sickness, there are a few things you can do to manage it. One strategy is to avoid the smells that bother you as much as possible. If the smell of coffee makes you feel nauseous, for example, you may want to steer clear of coffee shops or ask your partner to make their morning brew in another room.

Another tip is to keep some pleasant scents on hand to help mask any unpleasant odors. You could try using essential oils, such as peppermint or lavender, which are known for their calming and soothing properties. Just make sure to consult with your healthcare provider before using any essential oils during pregnancy.

In conclusion, a heightened sense of smell can be an early sign of pregnancy. It can make certain smells more noticeable and even trigger nausea. While it can be challenging to deal with, there are strategies you can use to manage it and make your pregnancy journey a little more comfortable.

Acne Breakouts

Acne breakouts and skin changes are common occurrences in early pregnancy due to hormonal changes. These hormonal fluctuations can lead to an increase in oil production, which can clog pores and result in the development of acne. Additionally, the increased blood flow and circulation during pregnancy can cause the skin to appear flushed or blotchy.

It is important to note that not all women will experience acne breakouts during pregnancy, and the severity can vary from person to person. Some women may only experience mild breakouts, while others may have more severe acne. The exact cause of these breakouts is not fully understood, but hormonal changes are believed to play a significant role.

To manage acne breakouts during pregnancy, it is important to maintain a gentle skincare routine. Avoid using harsh or abrasive products that can irritate the skin further. Instead, opt for gentle cleansers and moisturizers that are specifically formulated for sensitive skin. It is also advisable to avoid picking or popping any acne lesions, as this can lead to scarring.

In some cases, a dermatologist may recommend topical treatments that are safe for use during pregnancy, such as benzoyl peroxide or glycolic acid. However, it is crucial to consult with a healthcare provider before using any new skincare products or medications during pregnancy.

In addition to acne breakouts, hormonal changes during pregnancy can also cause other skin changes. Some women may notice an increase in pigmentation, particularly in areas such as the linea nigra (a dark line that forms on the abdomen) and the underarms. These changes are typically temporary and will fade after pregnancy.

In conclusion, hormonal changes in early pregnancy can lead to acne breakouts and skin changes. It is important to maintain a gentle skincare routine and consult with a healthcare provider for any concerns or questions regarding skincare during pregnancy.

Changes in Libido

During early pregnancy, many women experience changes in their libido, or sexual desire. This can be attributed to the hormonal fluctuations that occur in the body. The surge of hormones, such as estrogen and progesterone, can have a significant impact on a woman's sex drive.

For some women, these hormonal changes may result in an increase in libido, leading to a heightened desire for sexual intimacy. On the other hand, some women may experience a decrease in libido, feeling less interested in sex than usual. These changes in libido can vary from woman to woman and even from pregnancy to pregnancy.

It's important to remember that these changes are normal and temporary. The fluctuating hormones during early pregnancy can affect different women in different ways. Some women may find that their libido returns to normal as their pregnancy progresses, while others may continue to experience fluctuations throughout the entire pregnancy.

If you're experiencing changes in your libido during early pregnancy, it's essential to communicate openly with your partner and healthcare provider. Discussing your feelings and concerns can help both you and your partner understand and support each other during this time of transition.

In addition to hormonal changes, other factors such as fatigue, morning sickness, and physical discomfort may also contribute to changes in libido. It's important to listen to your body and prioritize self-care during this period. Engaging in open and honest communication with your partner can help ensure that both of your needs are met and that you navigate these changes together.

- Communicate openly with your partner about your changing libido and any concerns you may have.
- Take time for self-care and prioritize rest and relaxation.
- Explore alternative ways to connect with your partner, such as cuddling or non-sexual intimacy.
- Experiment with different positions or activities that may be more comfortable during pregnancy.
- Consult with your healthcare provider if you have any specific concerns or questions about your libido during pregnancy.

Abdominal Bloating

Abdominal bloating and gas are common early pregnancy symptoms that many women experience. This discomfort can be attributed to hormonal changes and the expanding uterus putting pressure on the digestive system. As a result, pregnant women may feel bloated and gassy, which can cause discomfort and even pain.

To alleviate these symptoms, there are several strategies that can be helpful. First and foremost, it is important to maintain a healthy and balanced diet. Avoiding foods that are known to cause gas, such as beans, cabbage, and carbonated drinks, can help reduce bloating. Instead, opt for foods that are rich in fiber, such as fruits, vegetables, and whole grains, as they can aid in digestion and prevent constipation.

In addition to dietary changes, it is also recommended to eat smaller meals throughout the day instead of large, heavy meals. This can help ease the burden on the digestive system and prevent excessive bloating. Drinking plenty of water and staying hydrated is also crucial in maintaining proper digestion and reducing bloating.

Regular exercise, such as walking or gentle yoga, can also be beneficial in relieving abdominal bloating. Physical activity promotes healthy digestion and can help alleviate gas and bloating. It is important to consult with a healthcare provider before starting or continuing any exercise routine during pregnancy.

If abdominal bloating persists or is accompanied by severe pain, it is important to seek medical advice. While bloating is a common symptom of early pregnancy, it can also be a sign of other underlying conditions. A healthcare provider can evaluate the symptoms and provide appropriate guidance and treatment if necessary.

Increased Basal Body Temperature

Tracking your basal body temperature (BBT) can be a useful tool in detecting early pregnancy. Basal body temperature refers to your body's temperature at rest, and it can fluctuate throughout your menstrual cycle. During ovulation, your BBT typically rises slightly, and if it remains elevated for more than two weeks, it could be an indication of pregnancy.

By monitoring your BBT daily and charting the changes, you may notice a small increase in temperature that persists beyond your usual luteal phase. This rise in BBT occurs due to the hormone progesterone, which is released after ovulation and helps prepare the uterus for pregnancy.

To track your BBT accurately, you will need a basal body thermometer, which is more sensitive than regular thermometers. It is essential to take your temperature first thing in the morning before engaging in any activity, as physical movement can affect your BBT. Make sure to record your temperature consistently at the same time every day.

Creating a BBT chart can help you identify patterns and changes in your temperature over time. You can use a table or a graph to plot your daily temperatures. Look for a sustained increase in BBT for at least 18 days, as this may indicate pregnancy. However, it is important to note that BBT alone cannot confirm pregnancy, and other early signs should also be considered.

If you suspect you may be pregnant based on your BBT chart, it is advisable to take a home pregnancy test or consult with a healthcare professional for confirmation. They can provide further guidance and support throughout your pregnancy journey.

Heightened Sensitivity to Smells

During early pregnancy, many women experience a heightened sensitivity to smells, which can be quite surprising. Suddenly, everyday scents that were once pleasant or neutral can become overwhelming and even nauseating. This sensitivity to smells is often linked to the hormonal changes that occur in the body during pregnancy.

Have you ever walked into a room and been hit by a strong smell that no one else seems to notice? Well, that's what it feels like for some pregnant women. It's as if their sense of smell has been turned up to maximum volume, making even the slightest scent feel overpowering.

This heightened sensitivity to smells can be both a blessing and a curse. On one hand, it can make certain foods or odors unbearable, leading to nausea or even vomiting. On the other hand, it can also make pleasant smells even more enjoyable. Some women find that they have a newfound appreciation for the aroma of fresh flowers or the scent of their partner's cologne.

So, why does this happen?

During pregnancy, hormonal changes can affect the olfactory system, which is responsible for our sense of smell. The increase in estrogen levels can make the olfactory receptors more sensitive, causing even the faintest of smells to be amplified. This heightened sensitivity to smells is thought to be a protective mechanism, helping pregnant women avoid potentially harmful substances.

How can you manage it?

If you're experiencing a heightened sensitivity to smells during early pregnancy, there are a few things you can do to manage it:

- Avoid strong odors: Try to stay away from strong-smelling foods, perfumes, cleaning products, and other substances that trigger your sensitivity.
- Keep a pleasant scent nearby: Carrying a small bottle of essential oil or a scented handkerchief with a soothing scent can help mask unpleasant smells and provide a comforting aroma.
- Take breaks outside: Fresh air can help clear your senses and provide relief from overwhelming smells. Take short walks outside whenever you feel overwhelmed.
- Stay hydrated: Drinking plenty of water can help dilute the concentration of smells in your nasal passages and reduce their intensity.
- Talk to your healthcare provider: If your sensitivity to smells is causing significant distress or interfering with your daily life, it's important to discuss it with your healthcare provider. They may be able to provide additional guidance or recommend strategies to help manage your symptoms.

Remember, every pregnancy is different, and not all women will experience a heightened sensitivity to smells. However, if you find yourself suddenly repelled by certain scents or feeling an intense attraction to others, it could be a sign that you're expecting.

Cramping

Cramping is a common early sign of pregnancy that can cause discomfort and concern for many women. It occurs as the uterus begins to expand and the ligaments stretch to accommodate the growing fetus. While cramping can be alarming, it is usually mild and not a cause for alarm.

The cramping sensation is often described as similar to menstrual cramps and can occur in the lower abdomen. It may be accompanied by a dull ache or a feeling of pressure. Some women may also experience cramping in the lower back or pelvic area.

These cramps are typically caused by the hormonal changes that occur in early pregnancy. As the uterus expands, it puts pressure on the surrounding muscles and ligaments, leading to cramping. Additionally, the increase in blood flow to the pelvic area can also contribute to cramping.

It's important to note that while mild cramping is normal, severe or persistent cramping should be evaluated by a healthcare provider. This could be a sign of an ectopic pregnancy or other complications.

To alleviate cramping, there are several self-care measures that can be taken. These include:

- Resting and taking breaks throughout the day
- Applying a heating pad or warm compress to the lower abdomen
- Taking a warm bath
- Engaging in gentle exercises, such as walking or prenatal yoga
- Practicing relaxation techniques, such as deep breathing or meditation

It's important to listen to your body and take care of yourself during this time. If you have any concerns or questions about cramping or any other symptoms you may be experiencing, it's always best to consult with your healthcare provider.

Back Pain

Back pain is a common symptom experienced by many women in early pregnancy. It can range from mild discomfort to more severe pain, and can be caused by a variety of factors. One of the main causes of back pain in early pregnancy is hormonal changes. During pregnancy, the body produces a hormone called relaxin, which helps to loosen the ligaments in the pelvic area in preparation for childbirth. However, this hormone can also affect the ligaments and muscles in the back, leading to pain and discomfort.

In addition to hormonal changes, posture adjustments can also contribute to back pain in early pregnancy. As the uterus grows and the baby develops, the woman's center of gravity shifts forward, causing the lower back to curve more than usual. This change in posture can put strain on the muscles and ligaments in the back, leading to pain and discomfort.

To alleviate back pain in early pregnancy, there are several things that women can try. Maintaining good posture throughout the day can help to reduce strain on the back. This includes sitting up straight, using a supportive chair, and avoiding standing or sitting for long periods of time. Engaging in gentle exercises, such as walking or swimming, can also help to strengthen the muscles in the back and alleviate pain. Additionally, using a supportive pillow while sleeping and wearing supportive shoes can provide extra comfort and support.

Changes in Taste

During early pregnancy, many women experience changes in their taste preferences and sensations. These changes can manifest as a metallic or bitter taste in the mouth, which can be an early sign of pregnancy.

One possible explanation for this change in taste is the hormonal fluctuations that occur during pregnancy. The increase in hormones, such as estrogen and progesterone, can alter the way taste buds perceive flavors. This can lead to a heightened sensitivity to certain tastes or a complete aversion to foods that were once enjoyed.

Some women may find that previously favorite foods now taste off-putting or even repulsive. On the other hand, they may develop cravings for specific foods that they never had an interest in before. These changes in taste can be quite surprising and may catch women off guard, especially if they are not aware of the early signs of pregnancy.

It is important to note that changes in taste can vary from woman to woman. While some may experience a metallic or bitter taste, others may notice a sweet or sour taste in their mouth. These taste changes are usually temporary and tend to subside as the pregnancy progresses.

If you suspect that you may be pregnant and are experiencing changes in taste, it is always a good idea to take a pregnancy test or consult with your healthcare provider for confirmation. They can provide you with the necessary guidance and support throughout your pregnancy journey.

Changes in Cervical Mucus

Changes in cervical mucus texture and consistency can be an important indicator of early pregnancy. During the menstrual cycle, the cervix produces different types of mucus that can vary in appearance and feel. Understanding these changes can help women identify potential signs of pregnancy.

In the early stages of pregnancy, cervical mucus may undergo noticeable transformations. One common change is an increase in the amount of mucus produced. Women may notice a greater presence of cervical mucus than usual, which can be a sign that conception has occurred.

Additionally, the texture and consistency of cervical mucus may change during early pregnancy. Prior to ovulation, cervical mucus tends to be sticky and thick, making it difficult for sperm to penetrate. However, in early pregnancy, the mucus becomes thinner and more slippery, resembling egg whites. This change in texture creates a more favorable environment for sperm to travel through the cervix and reach the egg for fertilization.

Monitoring changes in cervical mucus can be done by observing the mucus on toilet paper or by performing a self-check. Women can use their fingers to assess the texture and consistency of the mucus. By tracking these changes over time, women may be able to detect early signs of pregnancy before a missed period or positive pregnancy test.

It is important to note that changes in cervical mucus alone are not definitive proof of pregnancy. Other factors, such as hormonal fluctuations or certain medications, can also affect cervical mucus consistency. Therefore, it is recommended to consider changes in cervical mucus alongside other early pregnancy symptoms for a more accurate assessment.

- Increased amount of cervical mucus
- Thinner and more slippery texture
- Resembles egg whites

If you suspect you may be pregnant, it is always best to consult with a healthcare professional for a proper diagnosis and guidance on next steps.

Heightened Emotions

During early pregnancy, many women experience heightened emotions, including increased sensitivity and mood swings. These emotional changes are a result of the hormonal fluctuations that occur as the body adjusts to the presence of a growing fetus.

One of the main hormones responsible for these emotional changes is progesterone. Progesterone levels rise significantly during early pregnancy, and this can have a profound effect on a woman's mood and emotions. Some women may find themselves feeling more emotional than usual, with mood swings that can range from feeling elated one moment to tearful the next.

In addition to the hormonal changes, the physical and psychological adjustments that come with early pregnancy can also contribute to heightened emotions. The realization of being pregnant and the anticipation of the changes that lie ahead can lead to a mix of excitement, anxiety, and even fear. It's important to remember that these emotions are completely normal and part of the journey of becoming a mother.

It's also worth noting that every woman's experience of heightened emotions during early pregnancy can be different. Some may find themselves more sensitive to everyday stressors, while others may have more intense mood swings. It's essential to have a support system in place, whether it's a partner, family, or friends, who can provide understanding and empathy during this time.

To cope with heightened emotions, it can be helpful to engage in self-care activities that promote relaxation and stress reduction. This can include practices such as meditation, deep breathing exercises, gentle exercise, and finding time for activities that bring joy and calmness. It's also important to communicate openly with your healthcare provider about any concerns or emotional challenges you may be experiencing.

In conclusion, heightened emotions, including increased sensitivity and mood swings, are common in early pregnancy. These emotional changes are a result of hormonal fluctuations and the adjustments that come with the journey of pregnancy. Remember to take care of yourself and seek support when needed.

Cravings for Certain Foods

Cravings for certain foods are a common occurrence during early pregnancy. Many women experience intense desires for specific types of food that they may not have had an interest in before. These cravings can range from sweet and salty snacks to unusual combinations of flavors. While the exact cause of food cravings during pregnancy is not fully understood, hormonal changes are believed to play a significant role.

One theory suggests that hormonal fluctuations, particularly changes in estrogen and progesterone levels, can impact the areas of the brain that regulate appetite and cravings. These hormonal changes can lead to an increase in certain neurotransmitters, such as dopamine, which is associated with pleasure and reward. As a result, pregnant women may develop strong cravings for foods that provide a sense of satisfaction and comfort.

It's important to note that cravings for certain foods during pregnancy should not be ignored. They can be a signal that your body is lacking specific nutrients. For example, a craving for citrus fruits may indicate a need for vitamin C, while a craving for red meat could be a sign of low iron levels. It's essential to listen to your body's cues and try to satisfy these cravings in a healthy way.

To satisfy food cravings healthily, it's important to make nutritious choices. Instead of indulging in unhealthy processed foods or sugary treats, opt for nutrient-dense alternatives. For example, if you're craving something sweet, reach for a piece of fresh fruit or a smoothie made with natural ingredients. If you're craving something salty, choose roasted nuts or seeds instead of chips or pretzels.

Additionally, it's crucial to maintain a balanced diet during pregnancy to ensure you and your baby are getting all the necessary nutrients. Incorporate a variety of fruits, vegetables, whole grains, lean proteins, and healthy fats into your meals. If you're unsure about meeting your nutritional needs, consult with a healthcare professional or a registered dietitian who can provide personalized guidance.

Remember, cravings for certain foods during early pregnancy are normal and can be managed in a healthy way. By listening to your body's signals and making nutritious choices, you can satisfy your cravings while supporting your overall health and the well-being of your baby.

Nasal Congestion

Nasal congestion and stuffiness are often associated with the common cold or allergies, but did you know that they can also be early signs of pregnancy? It may seem surprising, but hormonal changes during pregnancy can actually cause your nasal passages to become swollen and congested.

During pregnancy, the body produces higher levels of estrogen and progesterone, which can lead to an increase in blood flow to the mucous membranes in your nose. This increased blood flow can cause the tissues in your nasal passages to swell, resulting in that stuffy feeling and difficulty breathing through your nose.

Additionally, the hormonal changes can also cause an increase in the production of mucus, leading to a runny or stuffy nose. This can be particularly bothersome at night when you're trying to sleep, as it can make it harder to breathe comfortably.

While nasal congestion and stuffiness can be uncomfortable, there are some things you can do to help alleviate the symptoms. Using a humidifier in your bedroom can help add moisture to the air and reduce dryness in your nasal passages. Saline nasal sprays or rinses can also help to clear out any excess mucus and relieve congestion.

It's important to note that nasal congestion and stuffiness alone are not definitive signs of pregnancy, as they can also be caused by other factors such as allergies or sinus infections. However, if you're experiencing nasal congestion along with other early pregnancy symptoms, such as fatigue, breast tenderness, and a missed period, it may be worth considering taking a pregnancy test to confirm.

Remember, every woman's experience with pregnancy symptoms can vary, so it's always best to consult with your healthcare provider if you have any concerns or questions about your symptoms. They can provide you with personalized guidance and support throughout your pregnancy journey.

Changes in Saliva

During early pregnancy, some women may experience changes in the consistency and taste of their saliva. These changes can be attributed to the hormonal fluctuations that occur in the body.

One common change is an increase in saliva production, which can lead to a constant feeling of having a "watery mouth." This excessive saliva, known as hypersalivation or ptyalism, can be bothersome and uncomfortable for some women.

Additionally, the taste of saliva may also change during early pregnancy. Some women report a metallic or bitter taste in their mouth, which can be persistent throughout the day. This altered taste sensation is often attributed to the hormonal changes affecting the taste buds.

It is important to note that these changes in saliva are not experienced by all pregnant women, and the intensity of the symptoms can vary. If you are experiencing excessive saliva production or a change in taste that is causing discomfort, it is recommended to speak with your healthcare provider for guidance and support.

Increased Thirst

Increased Thirst

Increased thirst can be a surprising early sign of pregnancy that many women may not be aware of. It is believed that hormonal changes during pregnancy can affect the body's fluid balance, leading to an increased need for hydration. As the body works hard to support the growing fetus, it requires more water to maintain proper functioning.

During early pregnancy, the body experiences an increase in blood volume, which can lead to dehydration if not properly addressed. This can result in feelings of thirst and a constant need to drink water. It is essential for pregnant women to stay hydrated to support their overall health and well-being.

To stay hydrated during pregnancy, it is recommended to drink plenty of water throughout the day. Aim for at least eight to ten glasses of water daily. If plain water becomes boring, you can add a slice of lemon or cucumber for a refreshing twist. Additionally, consuming fruits and vegetables with high water content, such as watermelon and cucumber, can also contribute to your hydration levels.

It is important to note that excessive thirst, paired with other symptoms such as frequent urination and fatigue, could be a sign of gestational diabetes. If you are experiencing extreme thirst and other concerning symptoms, it is best to consult with your healthcare provider for a proper diagnosis and guidance.

Remember, staying hydrated is crucial during pregnancy to support your body's changing needs. Listen to your body and drink water whenever you feel thirsty. By maintaining proper hydration, you can help ensure a healthy pregnancy and support the well-being of both you and your baby.

Skin Darkening

During early pregnancy, hormonal changes can lead to various changes in the body, including skin darkening. This is a common occurrence and can affect different areas of the body, such as the linea nigra and underarms.

The linea nigra is a dark line that may appear on the abdomen during pregnancy. It typically runs from the pubic bone to the belly button and is caused by an increase in melanin production. This darkening of the skin is completely normal and usually fades after pregnancy.

In addition to the linea nigra, some women may also experience darkening of the underarms. This is known as acanthosis nigricans and is characterized by thickened, darkened skin in the armpit area. Hormonal changes during pregnancy can contribute to this condition, but it is also associated with insulin resistance. It is important to note that acanthosis nigricans can occur in non-pregnant individuals as well and may be a sign of an underlying medical condition.

If you notice any changes in your skin during pregnancy, it is always a good idea to consult with your healthcare provider. They can provide guidance and ensure that everything is progressing normally. It is also important to protect your skin from excessive sun exposure and use sunscreen to prevent further darkening.

Frequently Asked Questions

- **What are the early signs of pregnancy?**

  There are several early signs of pregnancy that women may experience before a missed period or positive pregnancy test. These signs include breast changes, increased urination, changes in vaginal discharge, spotting or light bleeding, changes in sense of smell, fatigue, morning sickness, food cravings and aversions, mood swings, constipation, headaches, dizziness, heightened sense of smell, acne breakouts, changes in libido, abdominal bloating, increased basal body temperature, heightened sensitivity to smells, cramping, back pain, changes in taste, changes in cervical mucus, heightened emotions, cravings for certain foods, nasal congestion, changes in saliva, increased thirst, and skin darkening.

- **What breast changes can occur in early pregnancy?**

  During early pregnancy, it is common to experience breast tenderness, swelling, and darkening of the nipples. These changes are due to hormonal fluctuations in the body.

- **Why do I need to urinate more frequently in early pregnancy?**

  Frequent urination is a possible early sign of pregnancy. Hormonal changes during pregnancy can affect the bladder, causing it to fill up more quickly and leading to the need to urinate more frequently.

- **How does vaginal discharge change in early pregnancy?**

  In early pregnancy, you may notice changes in vaginal discharge. It may increase in amount and have a different consistency than usual. This is a normal occurrence and is caused by hormonal changes in the body.

- **What is implantation bleeding?**

Implantation bleeding is a common early pregnancy symptom that may be mistaken for a light period. It occurs when the fertilized egg implants itself into the uterine lining. The bleeding is usually light and may last for a few days.

- **Why do I have a heightened sense of smell during early pregnancy?**

Many women experience a heightened sense of smell or aversion to certain odors in early pregnancy. This is believed to be due to hormonal changes in the body. Certain smells may trigger nausea or discomfort.

- **Why am I feeling extremely tired and fatigued in early pregnancy?**

Extreme tiredness and fatigue are common in early pregnancy. This is because hormonal changes can affect energy levels and the increased demands on the body during pregnancy.

- **What is morning sickness and how can I manage it?**

Morning sickness is a classic symptom of pregnancy. It is characterized by nausea and vomiting, usually occurring in the morning but can happen at any time of the day. To manage morning sickness, it is recommended to eat small, frequent meals, avoid triggers, stay hydrated, and get plenty of rest.

- **Why do I experience food cravings and aversions in early pregnancy?**

Many pregnant women experience strange food cravings and aversions in the early stages. These cravings and aversions are believed to be influenced by hormonal changes in the body. It is important to listen to your body's cravings but also maintain a balanced and healthy diet.

- **What causes mood swings during early pregnancy?**

Hormonal fluctuations during early pregnancy can lead to mood swings and emotional changes. It is normal to experience a range of emotions during this time. It is important to take care of your mental health and seek support if needed.

- **Why do I experience constipation in early pregnancy?**

Constipation is a common early pregnancy symptom. Hormonal changes can affect the digestive system, slowing down bowel movements and leading to constipation. It is important to stay hydrated, eat fiber-rich foods, and engage in regular physical activity to alleviate constipation.

- **What causes headaches in early pregnancy?**

Headaches in early pregnancy can be caused by hormonal changes and increased blood volume. It is important to stay hydrated, practice relaxation techniques, and manage stress to help alleviate headaches.

- **Why do I feel dizzy and lightheaded in early pregnancy?**

Feelings of dizziness and lightheadedness can occur in early pregnancy due to hormonal changes and increased blood flow. It is important to avoid sudden movements, stay hydrated, and get up slowly from a sitting or lying position to manage dizziness.

- **Why do I have acne breakouts in early pregnancy?**

Hormonal changes in early pregnancy can lead to acne breakouts and changes in the skin. It is important to maintain a good skincare routine and consult with a healthcare professional for safe acne treatment options during pregnancy.

- **How do hormonal changes affect libido in early pregnancy?**

Hormonal changes can have varying effects on libido in early pregnancy. Some women may experience an increase in libido, while others may experience a decrease. It is important to communicate with your partner and prioritize open and honest discussions about intimacy during this time.

- **Why do I experience abdominal bloating and gas in early pregnancy?**

Abdominal bloating and gas are common early pregnancy symptoms. Hormonal changes can affect digestion and lead to increased gas and bloating. It is important to eat smaller, more frequent meals, avoid gas-producing foods, and engage in gentle physical activity to alleviate these symptoms.

- **How can tracking basal body temperature help detect early pregnancy?**

Tracking basal body temperature can help detect early pregnancy as there is a slight increase in temperature after ovulation and implantation. By monitoring changes in basal body temperature over time, you may be able to identify patterns that indicate pregnancy.

- **Why do I have cramping in early pregnancy?**

Mild cramping can occur in early pregnancy as the uterus expands and ligaments stretch to accommodate the growing fetus. It is important to differentiate between normal cramping and severe or persistent pain, which may require medical attention.

- **What causes back pain in early pregnancy?**

Back pain in early pregnancy can be caused by hormonal changes, posture adjustments, and the growing uterus putting pressure on the lower back. Practicing good posture, engaging in gentle exercises, and using supportive pillows can help alleviate back pain.

- **Why do I experience changes in taste during early pregnancy?**

Changes in taste, such as a metallic or bitter taste, can be an early sign of pregnancy. Hormonal changes can affect the taste buds and alter the perception of flavors. These changes are usually temporary and subside as the pregnancy progresses.

- **How does cervical mucus change in early pregnancy?**

In early pregnancy, cervical mucus texture and consistency can change. It may become thicker, stickier, or have a different appearance than usual. These changes are influenced by hormonal fluctuations and can be used as a potential indicator of early pregnancy.

- **Why do I have nasal congestion in early pregnancy?**

Nasal congestion and stuffiness can be an early pregnancy symptom. Hormonal changes can cause the blood vessels in the nasal passages to swell, leading to congestion. Using saline nasal sprays and maintaining a humid environment can help alleviate nasal congestion.

- **What changes occur in saliva during early pregnancy?**

Some women may experience changes in saliva consistency and taste in early pregnancy. It may become thicker or have a different taste than usual. These changes are believed to be influenced by hormonal fluctuations.

- **Why do I feel increased thirst in early pregnancy?**

Increased thirst can be an early sign of pregnancy. Hormonal changes can affect fluid balance in the body, leading to increased thirst. It is important to stay hydrated by drinking plenty of water throughout the day.

- **How do hormonal changes cause skin darkening in early pregnancy?**

Hormonal changes during early pregnancy can cause skin darkening, such as the formation of the linea nigra (a dark line on the abdomen) and darkened underarms. These changes are temporary and usually fade after pregnancy.

Have Questions / Comments?

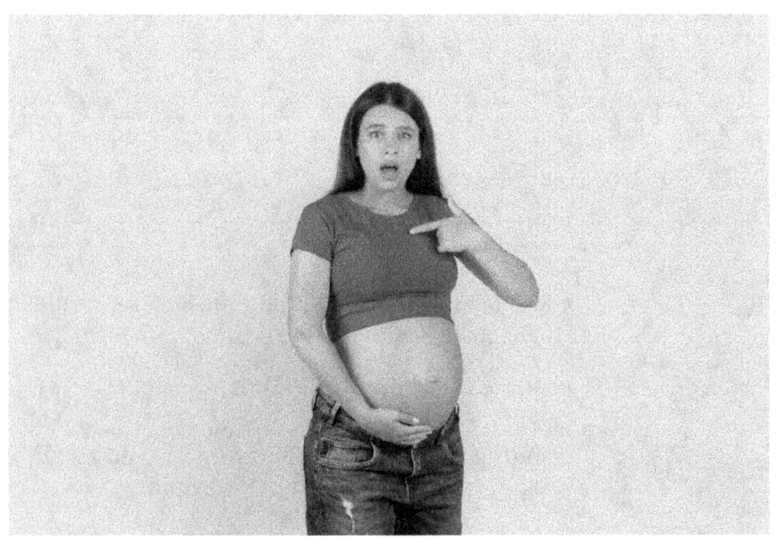

This book was designed to cover as much info as possible but I know I have probably missed something, or some new amazing discovery that has just come out.

If you notice something missing or have a question that I failed to answer, please get in touch and let me know. If I can, I will email you an answer and also update the book so others can also benefit from it.

Thanks For Being Awesome :)

Submit Your Questions / Comments At:
Get In Touch Babydreamers.net

Get How To Be A Super Mom
100% FREE

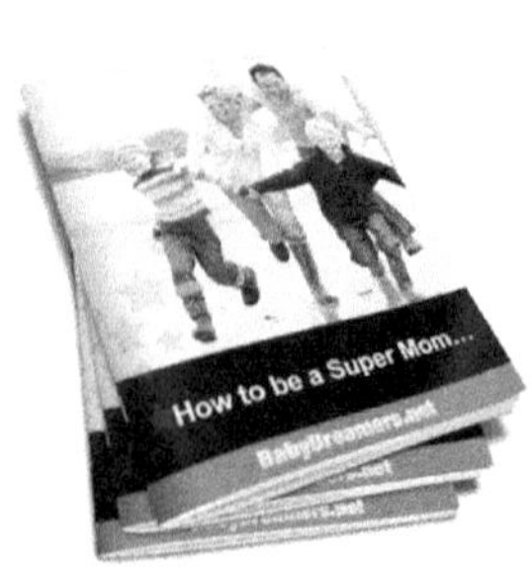

For being one of our amazing readers, we would love to offer you another book we have created, 100% free.

Being a mom is probably the most important job in the world – we've all heard that, and it's true. You're bringing up the next generation of wonderful, intelligent, loving, creative, responsible people.

We all want to be Super Mom and to be everything and do everything, but it this possible?

Being a Super Mom is possible, but you have to learn how to empower yourself to be the kind of Super Mom that you feel you need to be, keeping in mind that the title Super Mom doesn't mean the same thing to everyone.

<u>Get How to be a Super Mom For Free</u>